Quick-Easy Natural Colon-Blood Cleansing

"A simple cleanse using fruits, vegetables, and nutrients."

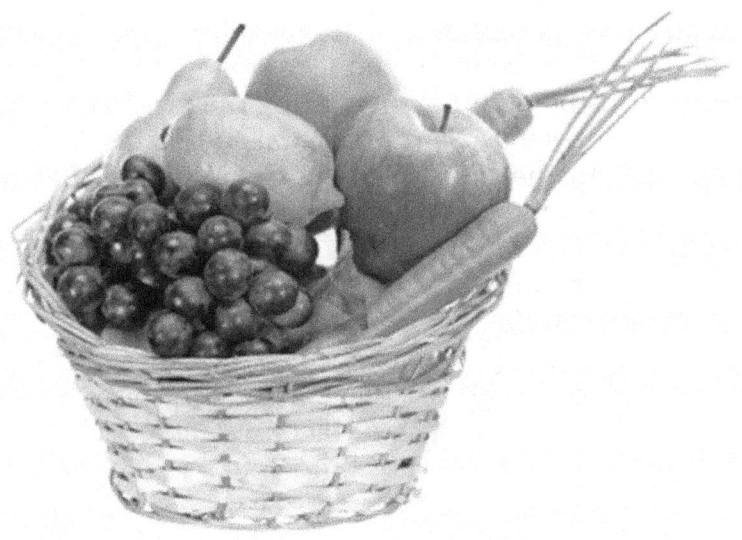

By Rudy S. Silva, Natural Nutrition

Quick-Easy Natural Colon-Blood Cleansing © 2012, by
Rudy S. Silva, Natural Nutritionist

ISBN-13:978-1481100809
ISBN-10:1481100807

Disclaimer and Terms of Use: The Author and Publisher has strived to be as accurate and complete as possible in the creation of this book, notwithstanding the fact that he does not warrant or represent at any time that the contents within are accurate due to the rapidly changing nature of the Internet. While all attempts have been made to verify information provided in this publication, the Author and Publisher assumes no responsibility for errors, omissions, or contrary interpretation of the subject matter herein. Any perceived slights of specific persons, peoples, or organizations are unintentional. In practical advice books, like anything else in life, there are no guarantees of income made. All readers are advised to seek services of competent professionals in the medical field

Your doctor or health provider should confirm any information given here. This information should not be taken as medical advice or treatment. This e-book is for information and educational purposes only.

Printed in the United States of America

Table of Contents

Introduction What To Expect From This e-Book

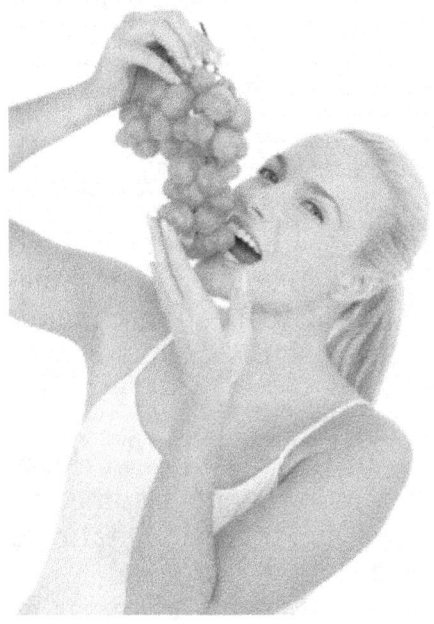

"You can do this body cleanse for three to five days."

Body Toxins Eliminated

One of the first steps to take when you have decided that you want to do something about your health is to do a colon and blood cleanse.

Not only should you do this cleanse to improve your health, but also when you fall ill to any disease as simple as constant mucus flow, skin eruptions or to a deadly disease as cancer.

When you do this cleanse, you pull toxins out of your individual cells, blood stream, stomach, small intestines, colon and every part of your body. When you have toxins in your blood and in your colon, it is hard for the toxins in your cells and lymph liquid to move out quickly into your blood, to be neutralized and eliminated by your liver and kidney.

Body toxins result in inflammation and mucus accumulation throughout your body. Your body is always trying to find a way to deal with your toxins, so it uses your channels of elimination – kidney, colon, lungs, skin, and liver - to get rid of them.

When your colon is overworked and filled with toxins, your body will eliminate body toxins through the other channels of elimination. Toxins will go to the kidney, lungs, liver, and skin. When toxins stay too long in these channels of elimination they cause inflammation, disease and sluggish function in these channels.

Toxins that remain in the cells and in the lymph liquid give rise to an acidic environment leading to an acid body, cardiovascular, cancer and other debilitating diseases.

The accumulation of toxic matter, in your body, gives rise to congestion such as mucus accumulation in your nose, sinus, throat, chest, and lungs. And this congestion is reflected in conditions such as sinus problems, bronchitis, colitis, asthma, acne, eczema, hives and many other skin disorders.

Benefits of This Colon and Blood Cleanse

By doing the colon and blood cleanse outline here, you can expect to gain a feeling of renewal. Toxins place a heavy load on your immune system and take a lot of energy to store and hide them in your body.

If you have some extra weight, you will lose a couple of pounds. This cleanse expels toxins and excess water all of which has some weight.

Acid body

This cleanse will give you a start on changing your body from an acid state to an alkaline state. You most likely have an acid body, since most people do. An acid body is where illness thrives, and you should make an effort to make your body more alkaline. Bacteria and all sorts of pathogens dislike an alkaline body. Various illnesses do not enjoy an alkaline body.

Once you complete the cleanse, information is provided so that you have a firm understanding on what you need to know to continue moving your body to an alkaline condition.

In the chapters of Body Cycles, you will discover how you can eat so that your body goes through a detoxification cycle each day. This cycle will help you to lose weight and to reduce the toxin load your body has to deal with every day.

1: Preparing For Colon-Blood Cleanse

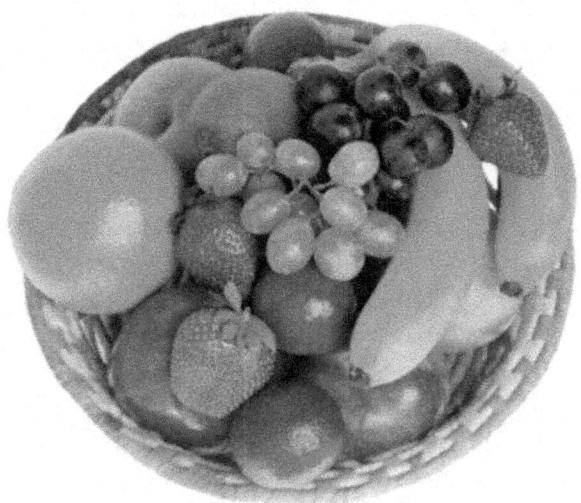

What the seven-day blood and colon cleanse does for you is:

- helps to remove toxins from your entire body
- provides nutrients to restore normal cell function
- cleanses the blood of toxins
- removes hardened waste or mucus that accumulates along colon walls
- removes excess mucus from your body
- gives you a feeling of well being
- improves your immune system

This cleanse consists of eating,

- fresh fruits
- fruit juices
- vegetables
- vegetable juices
- steamed vegetables

- herbal teas
- special nutrients

Special Nutritional Formulations

The best time for this cleanse is at the end of spring or early summer, when there are a lot of fresh fruits and vegetables. But, this cleanse can be done at any time. Doing this cleanse twice a year will give you great health benefits. And, you can do it during the week or whatever days you want.

You can also use steamed vegetable, but use a combination of steamed and fresh. Steamed vegetables help to clean your colon walls. Steam them for a few minutes, since certain nutrients evaporate or remain in the liquid.

Using herb teas will also enhance this cleanse. The herbal teas you should use are to help detoxify and cleanse the blood.

Here is a partial list of the foods you need to eat and, of course, a mixture and variety of different colors are best. Eating and using those fruits and vegetables that are grown locally is best, but you will find that what you use will come from other localities and this
is still ok.

Try buying and using organically grown fruits and vegetables. These can be found in health-food stores or at farmer's markets. The reason for using is organics is that non-organic produce is typically pesticide sprayed and these pesticides are quite toxic to your body. It doesn't make sense to eat toxic produce while trying to detoxify your body

Juices

Apple, Grape, Cherry, Orange, Lemons, Grapefruit, Pineapple, blueberry, blackberry, Cranberry, raspberry, combination of berries, Grapefruit, Carrot, Carrot-Apple, Carrot-Chlorophyll, Orange-Chlorophyll, Celery, Goats milk, raw milk.

Use a combination of different juices to get the benefit of their nutritional value. There are some juices that are not as sweet as others, so use them also.

Vegetables

Dark green lettuce, Beets, Carrots, Cucumbers, Cabbage, Tomatoes, Parsley, Onions, Spinach, Turnips, Asparagus, Garlic

Try to use those vegetables that you typically don't use. These vegetables will help you detoxify more. Stay away from the iceberg lettuce, since it has little nutritional value. You can use romaine and butter lettuce but try to use some of the others – the dark-green leafy ones.

Fruits

Watermelons, Cantaloupes, Casaba Melon, Strawberries, Cherries, Pears, Coconuts, Oranges, Peaches, Mangos, Apples, Bananas, Avocados

Herbal Teas

You can drink any herbal tea that you like.

Green tea, ginger tea, mint tea

2: Using Special Nutrients For Your Cleanse

Here are some special products or liquids that you can use to enhance this cleanse. Now, you don't have to use them, but they help give you a better cleanse. However, make sure you use at least the lemon juice, prune juice and the chlorophyll liquid.

Oxypowder, RubyReds, Chlorophyll, Lemon Juice, MSM, vitamin C powder, Prune Juice, Herbal teas

Oxypowder

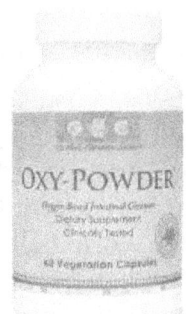

Oxypowder is a special formulated capsule designed to cleanse your colon. Unlike drugstore laxatives, it is not habit forming, but I recommend using it only until you use up all of the capsules in the bottle. The reason for using Oxypowder is it contains special nutrients – oxygenated magnesium, citric acid and organic germanium-132 – which liquefy and clear out sludge, mucus or fecal matter that has built up and accumulated along your colon walls or pockets and in the appendix area.

Since Oxypowder works with your stomach acid, you will benefit more by taking Oxypowder when you drink your lemonade drink in the morning. When you have a bowel movement, it will be liquid. This is not diarrhea.

Oxypowder converts hard stools into liquid, and this is the reason it can remove old embedded fecal matter from your colon. You may also have gas, since this is a byproduct of the chemical reaction of Oxypowder. This powder is not a laxative so you can use it knowing it is not habit forming.

Once you complete this cleanse with Oxypowder, your bowel movements should be regular. Keeping regular is important in keeping toxins to a minimum in your body. If you do not have regular bowel movements, stagnant fecal matter in your colon causes bad bacteria to multiply.

When toxins in your fecal matter stay against your colon walls longer than normal, they tend to be reabsorbed back into your blood. Toxins against your colon walls can weaken them, which can lead to various diseases.

Ruby Reds

Ruby Reds by Vitality is a special powder that containsall thee vitamins and minerals you need to keep healthy. It contains powders of many fruits and vegetables, fiber, probiotics, and digestive enzymes. You will enhance your blood

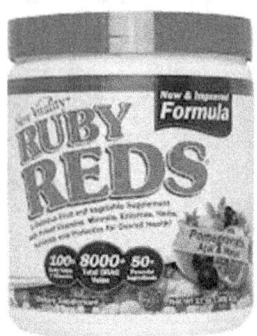 cleansing by using RubyReds powder, since you will be providing additional vitamins, minerals, phytonutrients, and antioxidants that are needed in your cells and in your lymph liquids to neutralize waste and acids. You will get all this from the juices you drink, but Ruby Reds gives you additional nutrients to cleanse out your body.

The way to use Ruby Reds is to add one capful of the powered into the juice that you will be drinking for the day. Or, if you make a smoothie, just add one capful to it. Ruby Reds has natural sugar so the taste of your drink with Ruby Reds will be enjoyable.

Lemons

Lemons are acidic when they first enter your mouth. In your mouth, minerals are secreted into your saliva to neutralize these acids. As the nutrients from the lemon reach your liver, they help to detoxify the liver. In the cells, lemon acids are changed into alkaline residues. As this alkaline residue gets back into the lymph liquid, it helps to neutralize any acid in the lymph liquid. Many toxins are in the form of acids, so these alkaline residues are very useful.

Chlorophyll

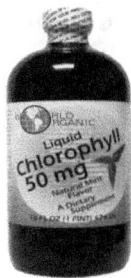 Use chlorophyll as a liquid. Chlorophyll is the blood source of plants. It is very similar in chemical structure to our blood. It will elevate your blood count and will work to neutralize and detoxify your body toxins. Using chlorophyll will reduce your body odor and stool smell. It gets into your blood and is used by all of your cells.

MSM

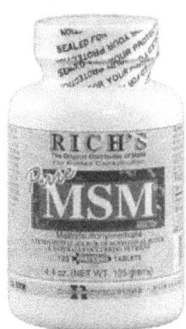 MSM or methylsulfonylmethane is organic sulfur. MSM is very critical in the body, since your body is composed of 1/3 MSM. After this cleanse, you should use MSM everyday – 2000-3000 mg minimum. MSM is considered the "Youth Supplement", since it will keep your cells and skin flexible. Cells need to be flexible and permeable so that nutrients can go in and out without any barriers.

For this cleanse MSM is very helpful. MSM is used inside the cell to neutralize free radicals and to tie up harmful proteins. In the cell membrane, it makes the membrane permeable, so that nutrients can go into the cell and toxins can move out of the cell. In effect, MSM keeps your cell membrane flexible and stops it from becoming leathery or hard, which prevents required chemicals from entering or leaving the cell.

One of the secrets of graceful aging is the effects that MSM has on your entire body. Your whole body benefits from MSM, since it keeps your skin and all tissue flexible and permeable, which is a necessity for good health.

In your colon, MSM leaves a film along the colon walls. This film prevents pathogen of various kinds from clinging to the walls. The result of this is they are flushed out with your stools.

MSM is also effective in promoting normal bowel movements. It activates peristaltic action. If you have not been having 1-3 bowel movements per day, this cleanse may help you become regular.

Herbal Teas

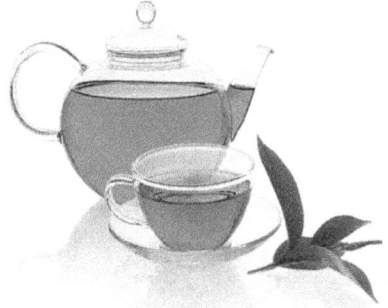

Herbs are considered food, but there are some interactions between them and some drugs. Herbs have powerful healing effects, since they contain numerous antioxidants, vitamins, minerals, and phytonutrients. When you eat or drink them, they work on the entire body, but also work more on specific organs or body systems. When used, they take a little longer to take effect compared to drugs, since the active ingredient in the herb is not as concentrated as in the drug.

The herbs you will be taking are to cleanse the blood of toxins that you will pull out of your cells and tissues. Also, your blood will be activated to be more active and move easier throughout your cardiovascular system. This helps you to have fewer toxic side effects, such as tissue pain, joint pain, nausea, stomach aches, or headaches.

You can mix your own herbs to create the tea you will use or you can buy it already made. Creating your own tea mixture is easier than you might think. You can get your individual herbs at some health or nutrition stores. The herbs that you find there will not be as fresh, active, and powerful as you need. You can go on the Internet and search for fresh herbs and for blood cleansing teas.

FRESH HERBS

From this list of herbs, pick out 3 or 4 of them to form your blood cleansing tea. These herbs help to detoxify, build, and activate your blood and lymph liquid.

- Yellow Dock Root
- Burdock Root
- Dandelion Root
- Red Clover
- Alfalfa
- Sarsaparilla
- Echinacea

Each day, drink one cup of this tea 1-2 hours after your lunch or dinner hour.

Here's how to prepare this blood cleansing tea.

Pour 1 1/4 cup of distilled water in a glass or porcelain container and heat to boil. Add one heaping tablespoon of herbs into the boiling water. Turn off the heat and let the herbal solution soak for 15 -20 minutes. The longer you leave this solution sit the stronger it will become. After soaking, pour the entire solution through a screen filter to remove the herbs. Now you can drink the herbal tea when it cools.

If you prefer to buy a blood cleansing herbal formula that works, do a Google search for, Blood Cleansing Formula

Food not to eat during clean

The foods not to eat during this cleanse are meat, fish, legumes, oils, fats of any kind, and carbohydrates. These types of foods will slow up your cleansing, since they take around 3 or more hours to digest. When eating juices, fruits and vegetable, they take only 1 -1 ½ hour to digest. This short digestion time helps you cleanse your body quickly by pulling toxins out of your body as you urinate, and as you have more frequent bowel movements.

3: Fruits and Vegetable Cleansing Diet

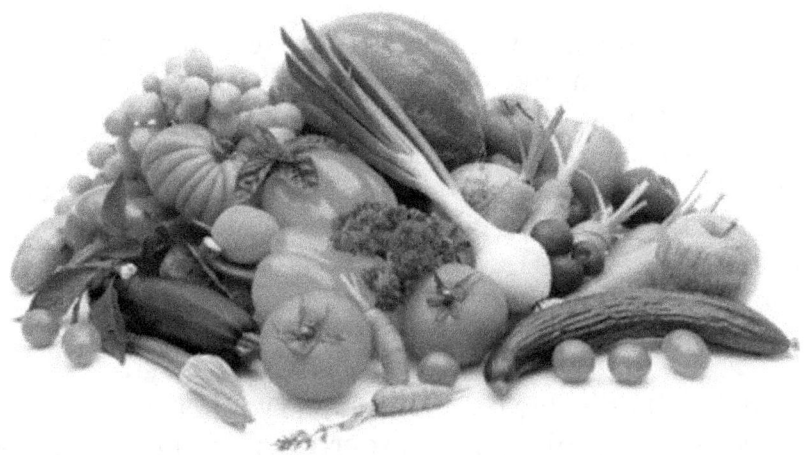

As you start this cleanse, keep in mind that you don't have to do what I have outlined here exactly. Each person is different as to what they have to do and what works for them, so chose the juices you like and set up the timeline that fits your life.

As you start this cleansing diet, you can develop symptoms that are uncomfortable. This may be headaches, running nose, gas, upset stomach, or a general feeling of "not feeling good." This is caused by toxins being stirred up throughout your body and your body looking for a way to get rid of them. Drinking the juices, teas, and special drinks will help you get past these feelings.

After a few days, these unpleasant symptoms will go away. If they don't, and they get worse then back off by one half of everything, you are doing and temporarily add a small amount of protein or carbohydrates to your diet. Then you can start your cleanse.

In the case of acne, you may see more acne breakouts as you start this cleanse. But, this also will stop, and you will see less and less breakouts, as you continue with your cleanse.

Things to do daily

Take a good supplement of calcium, magnesium and vitamin D. The magnesium and the vitamin D help you absorb more calcium. You can get the vitamin D your body needs by spending at least 30 minutes in the sun every day. But, using vitamin D with calcium is also a good idea. Taking calcium during body cleansing will help to neutralize toxic acidic waste.

Night Before the Cleanse

Around 6-8 pm the day before you start your cleanse, take 4 to 5 Oxypowder capsules. Oxypowder takes about 12 hours to activate your colon, so you will not need to go to the bathroom at night.

First day of Cleanse: Morning

When you wake, you will have a bowel movement that is watery. This is the Oxypowder at work.

Now, the first thing to do in the morning is take 3 – 4 capsules of Oxypowder and drink a chlorophyll drink – 1-2 oz of chlorophyll, the juice of one lemon, and the rest distilled or reverse osmosis water.

Around 1/2 hour later eat some fruit, such as watermelon, cantaloupes, or other fruit. In a thermos bottle – prepare 16 oz or more – pour in any type of juice. Add one capful of Ruby Reds and half to one teaspoon of powdered vitamin C.

Taking the Oxypowder will start your stomach, small intestine and colon cleanse. Oxypowder will liquefy your chime or fecal matter in your colon. It will also start to liquefy any fecal matter that has accumulated along your colon walls.

You will probably need to go to go to the bathroom around 2-3 times before noon. The sensations for a bowel movement will show up suddenly. But, when they do, you have a little of time before you needed to hurry to the bathroom. You can hold the bowel movement back, but plan on when you first feel that bathroom sensation to go to the bathroom first chance you get.

If you want less bowel movement activity, you should take only two Oxypowder capsules. The cleansing activity will be less, and if you plan to be at home, then you can take 4 or 5 capsules.

Then you can go to the bathroom immediately as needed.

Chlorophyll Drink

A chlorophyll drink will help to neutralize the toxins in your colon and the toxins that are in your body. This will help to minimize the toxic sickness feelings as you cleanse. The lemon will help to detox the liver and help it as it neutralizes toxins.

The watermelon or fruits put distilled water in your body, and they are diuretic, which pulls water out of your body and helps to cleanse the kidney. Also, the watermelon or fruits provide fiber to the colon, so that it can help the Oxypowder remove accumulated waste that attaches to the colon walls.

The vitamin C powder you put in the juice act as a preservative and prevent the juice from becoming rancid during the day.

Break time

An hour or so after breakfast, drink some of the juice you have prepared. You can drink this juice anytime you want during the day.

Dinner

Eat pieces of watermelon, cantaloupe, or other fruits and continue drinking your prepared juice. Prepare some steamed vegetables.

Take 3 capsules of Oxypowder as soon as you get home from work around 5-7 pm. I have found that Oxypowder during this time will not cause you to go to the bathroom at night, but each person is different. If you take more than 5 Oxypowder capsule, you may have to wake up during the night to have a bowel movement.

Eat one small cantaloupe and finish off your prepared juice drink, if you have not finished it. If it is after 5 pm, just dump the prepared juice drink that you did not drink. If you have finished, then drink a juice of another kind. Do not drink anything at least one hour or so before your bedtime.

Aside from having many bowel movements, you will also need to go to the bathroom to urinate.

Day Two of the Cleanse

Do the same thing you did on the first day.

If on the first day, you are having too many bowel movements, and it's interfering with your work; you can back off to two Oxypowder capsules in the morning and two at night. And if it is still too many bowel movements, then drop down to one capsule morning and night. You can experiment with how many Oxypowder capsules are right for you and your work schedule.

Third day of Cleanse

Do the same thing you did on the first day. But, now you should eat other fruits in the morning and throughout the day.

Also, start a vegetable drink such as carrot juice or a V8 type of drink. These V8 types of drinks are usually called veggie drinks.

If you are only doing a three day cleanse, then this is where you stop. But, don't start your normal eating, until the next day. The next day you want to start with the body cycle program. Start with only eating and drinking fruits and vegetables until noon.

Fourth day of Cleanse

On the fourth day, you will need to start your day early so that you have time to activate a bowel movement doing the following:

(You need to do this cleanse when you don't work or on a Saturday. You can plan your cleanse to start on Wednes - day so that this fourth day of cleansing is on Saturday.)

When you first wake up, here's what you do.

- Drink 2 cups, 8oz of prune juice half, then 1/2 hour later drink 8 oz of apple juice.

- If you do not have a bowel movement within the next ½ hour, then drink 8 oz more of apple juice.

After drinking the prune juice and apple juice, you will get an urgent call for a bowel movement. Be close to a bathroom at this time. You may have to go to the bathroom a couple of times in a short period; if not then you can go to work. But, at work, you will have to be ready to go to the bathroom frequently. If you cannot take this time, then it may be best to do this prune-apple juice cleanse Saturday, Sunday or on an off workday.

If you do the 3 day cleanse only, you can do this prune juice process the second day of your cleanse. If you are not doing the Oxypowder cleanse, then for sure do the prune juice process.

The prune juice one day cleanse is a powerful tool to purge out loose matter in the small intestine and in the colon. It activates the colon to produce strong peristaltic action to help clean out your colon. The prune and apple juice provide plenty of minerals and some vitamins to help neutralize acids in your body.

Fifty Day of Cleanse

Here's what to do on the fifth day.

- When you first wake up, take 3 capsules of Oxypowder. Do not drink the prune juices. Drink a chlorophyll drink or if you like you can add chlorophyll to carrot, veggie, or orange juice.

- Eat a bowl of fruit as much as you want.

- Repeat the fourth day of juices, fruits, and vegetables.

- Drink the following juices at these times:

1. Orange juice 1 quart as soon as you wake up
2. Grape juice 1 quart near noon time
3. Pineapple juice mid after noon
4. Orange juice around 6 pm
5. Drink these juices slowly over time. If you can't drink a quart at one time, drink at least 16 oz. Drinking this much juice at one time helps flush out your colon with liquid and aids you cleaning out your colon. You will have the urge to go to the bathroom right away, so be close to one.

6. If you can't drink that much juice at one time, drink the

juices slowly in sips. But, drink a glass or half a glass every 1/2 hour or every hour.

Sixth Day of Cleanse

- Repeat the third day. The use of prune juices was just for day4.

- The use of 1 quart of four different juices was only for the day 5.

- Eat fruits for breakfast and lunch, and drink the juices you like during the day.
- Eat a green salad at the end of the day with some apple cider vinegar

- Prepare a green salad with a variety of different fresh vegetables. You can add a small amount of flax seed oil, olive oil, and apple cider vinegar for your salad dressing. At the end of the day take 3 capsules of Oxypowder.

Seventh Day of Cleanse

- First thing in the morning, drink a green drink – chlorophyll and the juice of one lemon.

- Then, take 3 capsules of Oxypowder

- Eat plenty of raw green vegetable salads with olive oil, flaxseed oil, and apple cider vinegar.

- And drink fruit and vegetable juices throughout the day

- At the end of the day take another 3 Oxypowder capsules.

Final Cleansing Suggestions

There you have it, a seven-day fruit and vegetable juice fast. If you want to continue another day or so, continue eating fresh fruits and vegetables and drink a variety of juices, including orange, lemon, or grapefruit. If you want to do only a four or five day cleanse this is ok.

This colon and blood cleanse can be continued for a few more days, and if you follow the Body Cycles in the following chapters, you will be detoxifying your body every day.

This cleanse is designed to cleanse your colon and remove toxins from various parts of your body. It will also cleanse your blood and by drinking juices and eating fruits and vegetables, you are providing nutrients to your body, so that cells have the nutrients they need to regenerate properly.

Eat only fresh fruits and vegetables – slightly cook your vegetables, if you have colitis or for hemorrhoids. But, cooked vegetables lessen the nutritional value and decreases fiber benefit.

After your colon and blood cleanse, you now have a chance to start some new eating habits. The following chapters show you how to help your natural body cycles keep your body detoxified.

4: Kidney Cleanse

Cleansing different parts of the body and organs require different products, juices, or foods. Cleansing the kidney is done to remove small, medium or large kidney stones that may have form.

The first step in cleansing the kidney is to drink, first thing in the morning, a lemon-lime drink. It has been found that citrate in lemon, and lime juice helps keep those salts that form kidney stones in liquid form and thereby prevent stones from forming.

Studies at Duke University followed 12 kidney stone patients on lemonade therapy for four years. At the end, patients formed fewer kidney stones and these stones formed at a slower rate. During these four years, none of the patients required medical attention for kidney stones.

If you are prone to developing kidney stones, you should drink enough water or juice to produce around 2 liters of urine each day. If you have other medical issues or are on drugs, make sure you check with your doctor before using this lemonade cleanse or increasing your water intake.

Lemonade Kidney Cleansing Drink

Buy lemons, limes, and ½ ounce of cayenne powder.

In a blender squeeze one lemon and lime. After squeezing, with a spoon scrap out the remaining juice, pulp, and seeds, then add 8 – 12 oz of distilled water or reverse osmosis water.

Now, add just a pinch of cayenne powder. Start with just a pinch between the fingers so you can see how it affects you. If you make it too hot, you will not want to drink it. I recommend that you don't add any sugar, syrup, or honey. Just drink it plain. You will get used to this as you drink it.

Don't forget to add a couple of tablespoons or an oz of liquid chlorophyll to the lemonade drink. Give this drink the extra cleansing power.

To do a complete kidney cleanse, I recommend Dr Schulze "5 Day Kidney Cleanse." I have used this cleanse and it is an excellent cleanse. You can do this cleanse after you do the seven-day colon and blood cleanse. Or you might want to do both at the same time. Dr Schulze's kidney cleanse, may seem complicated, but it is not.

His cleanse calls for the above lemonade drink every morning. Then you drink 4 cups of his herbal tea during the day, in which you put some of his herbal extracts into a tea. And that's it. His kit also has herbal extracts to detoxify the colon.

This will cleanse out your colon and cause you to go to the bathroom frequently. But if you are doing the 7 day colon and blood cleanse, the Oxypowder will help you clean out your colon. You can save his detox herbal extract and do it in a couple of months.

5: Eating After Cleansing - Body Cycle 1

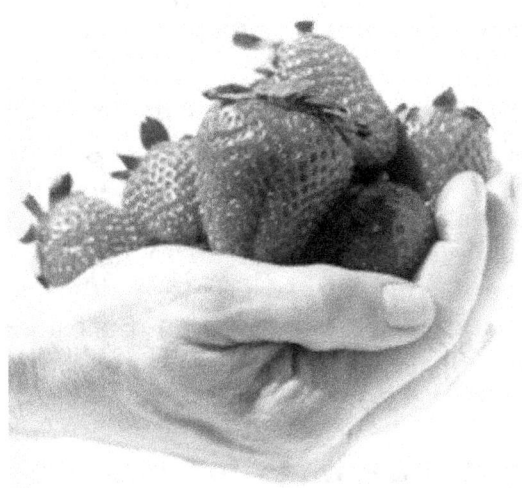

Now that you have completed your body cleanse, here is a way to eat so that you allow your body to keep cleansing itself using its natural body cycle.

Natural Body Cycles

Most of you are looking for ways to improve your health, lose weight, or get rid of an illness that you have. If you have acid reflux or heartburn, then you might be looking for a way to prevent it from coming back, after you have completed a colon cleanse

Here's some information that will help you achieve these results. It is called "Using the Natural Body Cycles" for achieving maximum health.

By learning how to assist your "Natural Body Cycles", you will be in tune with what your body is doing to maintain your health.

Getting in tune with your Natural Body Cycles requires a change in the way you eat. Since all of us are addicted to the way we eat, it is, sometimes, difficult to change these habits. But, if you are serious about what you want, this is the best information I have found that will give you good health.

Using this method to gain better health, you will experience side effects because you will be eliminating more body toxins and body wastes. The side effects may be headaches, stomach upsets, body pain, or similar types of symptoms. These conditions will not last and will disappear as you get rid of more toxins. So if you experience these side effects, don't let them stop you from moving forward on this eating pattern.

Here are the 3 natural body cycles:

Cycle 1 time period: 4 am to noon

This cycle is the time where your body is eliminating toxins, acids, wastes, and derby by urine, bowel movements, and other secretions.

Cycle 2 time period: noon to 8 pm

This is the time when your body should be taking in food and digesting

Cycle 3 time period: 8 pm to 4 am

This is the time your body is absorbing and using the food you have eaten during the noon to 8 pm period.

Here's how to use cycle 1:

Breakfast

During the elimination cycle, 4 am to noon, eat and drink only fruits and their juices or drink vegetable juices.

❖ For breakfast eat a bowl of fruit or have a fruit smoothie made with apple juice and fruits in season.

❖ Before noontime eat fruits as snack. Forty-five minutes before noon eat your last fruit. You can eat and drink all the fruits and juices you want up to noontime.

❖ Bananas, oranges, apricots, strawberries, melon, watermelons, apples, peaches, nectarines, and so on.

❖ Eat all melons together and not with other fruits and wait 1/2 hour before eating other fruits. Melons require their specific enzymes to be digested in your stomach, so other fruit eaten with melons will just sit in your stomach waiting to be digested.

By eating in this way you are assisting your body's elimination cycle. This helps your body to eliminate toxins and acids from your body and blood. It is these toxins and acids that make you sick and overweight.

Solid Food

Eating solid food for breakfast – eggs potatoes, rice, meat, cereal, milk, and so on - interfere with your body's elimination cycle and eventually leads to sickness and excess weight. It takes over 3 hours to digest heavy and solid food. The food you should be eating, in the morning, should digest quickly to help remove toxins, acids, and waste from your body that accumulates during the night.

Heavy food slows down the elimination of toxins from your body, and this causes more toxins to remain in your body. These stored toxins are converted to fat and acids. Acids are the main cause of most illnesses, so you want to have an alkaline body. Fruits and vegetables give you an alkaline body.

It takes up to 1 ½ hour or so to digest fruits and fruit juices. Because of this, they help to cleanse your body of waste, during the morning. Fruits are 70% water just like your body. So if you are not already having fruit and fruit juices for breakfast and snacks, start slowing changing your habits, if you want to lose weight and feel better.

Now, one other thing, don't eat fruits and juices with your lunch or dinner meals.

6: Natural Body Cycle 2

Again these cycles are:

Cycle 1 time period: 4 am to noon

This cycle is the time where your body is eliminating toxins, acids, wastes, and derby by urine, bowel movements, sweat, mucus, and other secretions.

Cycle 2 time period: noon to 8 pm

This is the time when your body should be taking in food and digesting

Cycle 3 time period: 8 pm to 4 am

During cycle 2 is time to eat solid food. What you eat has to be in alignment with what your stomach can do.

Here's how your stomach works. In generally, it can only digest one solid food at a time.

A solid food is one that does not contain 70% water, like fruits and vegetables do, and whose water has been eliminated by heat or other food processes, or cooked.

Your stomach can only work on one solid food at a time, so your lunch and dinner should have one solid food. A lunch can consist of chicken and a green salad, fish and a green salad, tuna and a green salad, shrimp and a green salad, beef and a green salad.

Mixing a protein meal with carbohydrates is giving the stomach two solid foods at the same time, which require different concentrations of digestive juices.

Giving the stomach more than it can handle interrupts the elimination cycle 1 and reduces the energy that you need for the elimination cycle.

Any eating habit that disrupts cycle 2, the eating and digestion cycle, affects the other cycles. Here's how you can help your body's cycle 2 to be more effective.

Eat only one solid food with vegetables during lunch or dinner. Lunch can be one meat or seafood with a fresh vegetable salad.

Limit the amount of water you drink during your eating. Excess water will dilute your digestive acids and slow down digestion of your food.

Eliminate drinking any sodas, coffee, tea or other drinks during your meals. If you need to clear your dry throat use a little water, which is a room temperature. Cold liquids will slow down your digestive processes.

Eating meals with more than one solid food such as meat and potatoes, chicken and rice, fish and rice, chicken and noodles, eggs and toast, cheese and bread will diminish the energy you need during the elimination cycle 1.

It is permissible to eat beef and chicken at the same time but not chicken and eggs or beef and nuts or chicken and beans. Eat the same type of protein at the same time but do not mix different proteins.

It's ok to eat different types of carbohydrates at the same time, with a salad, but not with protein, since carbohydrates digest easier than protein.

Eating a protein and a carbohydrate at the same time sets the stage for severe illness later in life. A protein requires acid for digestion and a carbohydrate requires alkaline juices for digestion.

This combination produces acid juices and alkaline juices at the same time. This combination produces water, which creates digestive juices that cannot fully digest either type of food.

In this case, the body produces more acid and more alkaline juices, which again are neutralized. The cycle continues until the food in your stomach starts to putrefy and ferment causing gas and acids. The gas causes belching, and the combination gas and acids can lead to acid reflux.

As foods turn into acids because of the putrefaction and fermentation process, this acid food spoils all the food in your stomach, causing undigested food to back flow up your esophagus and flow prematurely into your small intestine.

Food that is partially undigested becomes acidic, which affect the health of your colon, and when absorbed into your body is converted into fat and stored as a toxin your body.

In many cases the fermentation of food results in the production of alcohol and is similar to a person who drinks alcohol. There have been cases where people have been arrested for drunk driving and have never drank in their lives, and they wonder why they had a high blood-alcohol level.

Eating the right combinations of foods at mealtime helps to preserve your energy for the elimination cycle and prevents you from creating spoiled food in your stomach that is converted to acid waste.

It is this acid waste that results in illness and fat. This is the reason most people as they age come down with various illnesses that terminate their life early or gain excessive weight.

7: Natural Body Cycle 3

Cycle 3 is the assimilation cycle and is from 8pm to 4am. This is the time the food you have eaten during the day is assimilated, absorbed and distributed throughout your body through your blood.

Food that was eaten during cycle 2 that was combined and eaten properly will digest within 3 hours. Whereas food not combine properly, a meal consisting of protein and carbohydrates, will take up to 8 hours to pass through the stomach. During this time, your food will putrefy and ferment and become acidic. Under these conditions, you will not get a lot of nutrients from that meal.

Natural Body Cycle 3

Eat your last meal by 6-7 pm so that your food digests in your stomach by the time you go to bed. After three hours later, your food will have moved into your small intestine where it is ready for assimilation.

When you go to bed 3 hours after your last meal, the next 6 hours, until 4am, your body will be absorbing the food you have eaten the previous day.

Remember, anything you do different than what these cycles call for will disrupt them and cause them to become extended. When this happens, your food turns into acid, you don't absorb the value of your food, you lose energy and become tired, and over time, you gain weight and create serious illnesses.

Have you ever notices how everyone you know eventually comes down with some sickness, which require surgery or doctor's drugs. Think about it. Is this what you want happening to you? Just start changing your eating habits slowly and as time passes you will be doing more and more of what your body's natural cycles need.

8: Acid – Alkaline Body

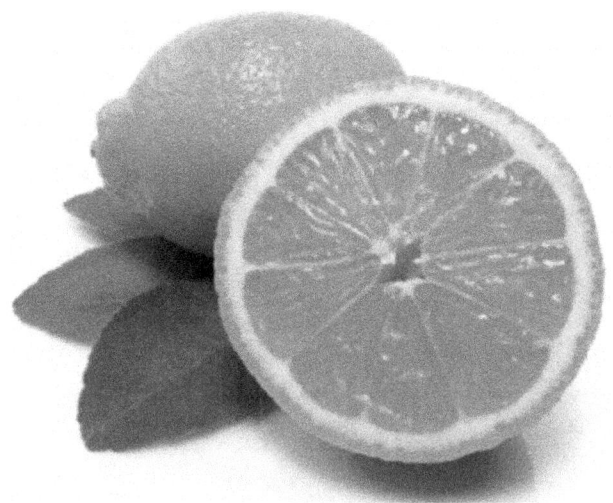

The principles in the Colon and Blood cleansing and the Body Cycles are designed to remove toxins from your body and to neutralize any remaining toxins with certain minerals. When this happens, you will be changing and keeping your body in an alkaline state. In this state, you can achieve the best health possible for your body.

Minerals

Moving your body more toward alkalinity is what will give you the best curative effects of fruits. An alkaline body prevents your body from becoming ill and forming deadly diseases, like joint problems, organ degradation, body pain, heart disease, or even cancer. If you are already sick, then all the chemicals inside fruits will help to revive you to better health. This is provided that your tissue damage has not gone beyond repair.

The minerals most importance in changing and maintaining your body in an alkaline condition are sodium, potassium, chloride, calcium, phosphorus, magnesium, and sulphur.

Now, how your body can become alkaline might become a little confusing at first because of the terms used, but let's break this down into small parts. First, we are going to be defining some terms, so we can then start talking the same language.

Acid Binding

There are certain minerals that are called acid binding. And, these are minerals we said are the most important ones in fruits, Sodium, potassium, chloride, calcium, phosphorus, magnesium, because they are acid binding.

What acid binding means is when you eat fruits with these minerals, they will seek out acids in your body and combine with them to neutralize them, by creating a new chemical called alkaline forming ash.

Alkaline Ash

After this alkaline forming ash has tied up an acid, it is carried to the kidney where it is expelled as urine.

Different reactions can occur when an acid binding mineral, like say sodium, encounters an acid. Of course, acids in the body are toxic, so the body has the priority of getting rid of them fast, since they can damage tissue and cause pain and disease.

Here is another path way of the acid binding mineral process, when it combines with an acid.

The Acid Binding Mineral Process

When you eat acid binding food, the blood carries it to the cells where it is oxidized, digested, or metabolized. The result of this digestion is a carbonic acid salt of alkaline minerals, which reacts with body acids and binds with them. In this process, a weak carbonic acid is created. Now, this weak carbonic acid is taken by the blood into your lungs where it is released as carbon dioxide and water.

If not all the acid toxins are captured by acid binding matter, the remaining acids can be neutralized by body stores of alkaline minerals. If you don't have a good store of alkaline minerals, then these acids will remain in your body creating disease. But, if you do have a good store of alkaline minerals, these minerals will find acids, capture them, and bind with them. Then these acids are routed out through your urine and out of your body.

So you can see the importance of getting a lot of alkaline minerals into your body. Without them, acids, which do not get bonded to alkaline minerals, would move back into body tissue and continue their body damage.

Alkaline Binding

Now, there are also minerals that become alkaline binding and these minerals are sulphur, chlorine, iodine, phosphorus, bromine, fluorine, copper, and silicon. It is these minerals that when digested by a cell will produce a salt that will bind with alkaline minerals. These minerals will be excreted through your urine. When alkaline minerals are bonded to an acid salt, the alkaline mineral is removed from your body and your body becomes more acidic, the condition you are trying to avoid.

Although you need to eat both foods that are acid binding or alkaline binding, you want to eat more of the acid binding food. This will keep your body slightly alkaline.

Keeping Healthy

One of the most important parts of health is keeping the lymph liquid around your cells clean and free of toxins. To do this you need to provide acid binding minerals to occupy the lymph liquid. These minerals remove the acids that accumulate in your lymph liquid and in all parts of your body tissue.

Body Detoxification

The highest priority of the body is to detoxify itself. This helps you to lose weight and to maintain normal weight. One of the best way to help your body detoxify is to provide minerals that bind with acids that are in the cells, tissues, organs, and muscles. What these minerals do is to pull out the toxins that are dispersed throughout your body.

These minerals have the ability to suck those acids out and bind with them. But, because not all body chemical reactions follow the same directions there are times that the acid does not take place.

With the help of the liver, which detoxifies the blood, the kidney removes impurities from the blood and the lungs. The lungs will remove the CO_2, which resulted from minerals or acid binding food.

Your body is constantly detoxifying itself. But, when it is over loaded with acid toxins from your lifestyle, a complete detox of your body may become impossible.

Where do Acid Toxins Come From?

So why is the body overloaded with toxins? Why can't the liver take care of these toxins? Your liver has the function to remove acid wastes from natural food that is created by food digestion and cell metabolism.

When your body encounters acid wastes, such as food enhancers, dyes, preservatives, pesticides, and the variety of additives, the liver does not know how to break them down and to make them harmless.

But, your body doesnot give up so easily, when it knows that the liver was not able to disintegrate food additives. What it does is it instructs calcium to bind with these toxic acids and to take them far away from the blood stream.

When calcium binds with acids, a calcium deposit can form in your teeth, and your joints as bone spurs, which grow in your feet or shoulders, vertebrae, or muscle tissue. These calcium deposits are very painful, and if you have ever experience them, you know how much.

Now, we have talked about acid toxins in the body that are brought in through food and the environment. But, there is another factor that creates acid in your body and this is emotions that are activated through life stresses, like work pressures, divorce, friendship problems, martial issues, and other similar problems. These emotional problems create acidic molecules, which embed themselves into your tissues just like food acids

Body Organs

All body organs function to rid the body of acid waste or toxins. Lack of acid binding food causes deterioration of the function of these organs. Each organ has a specific function in the elimination and neutralization of acid wastes and it does this in conjunction with acid binding food which are alkaline minerals.

In the next chapter is a list of the fruits that have the highest alkaline minerals, and the ones that you should be eating.

The percentage assigned to these fruits is based on fresh fruits that are organic and that are not cooked, canned or mixed with sugar. If they are cooked or otherwise processed in some fashion, this will reduce their effectiveness as an acid binding fruit. However, they will still be somewhat effective as acid binding food.

9: Acid Binding Fruits With Alkaline Minerals

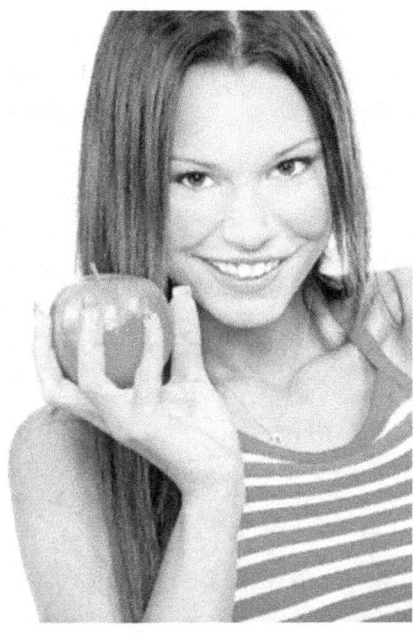

In the list below are fruits are acid binding food or alkaline minerals that create an acid binding salt your body used to neutralize acid wastes. Fruits above 50% in value are more acid binding, which means they will trap acid wastes better. You will want to eat and drink those fruits above 51%.

The fruits that are at 50% at are neutral. They are not acid binding nor alkaline binding.

Fruits below 50% are alkaline binding food and create more acid in your body.
You should eat and drink fruits from all these levels, but eat 80% of the fruits that are above 50%.

Here is the list of fruits to eat and drink in the order of priority.

1. Fruits at 100% Acid Binding – Best fruits To Eat And Drink Lemons, melons – any type, watermelon

2. Fruits at 93% Acid Binding – Great fruits To Eat And Drink Cantaloupes, dried dates, dried figs, limes, mango, papaya

3. Fruits at 87% Acid Binding – Still Great Fruits To Eat And Drink Kiwis, passion fruit, pineapples, raisins, umeboshi plums

4. Fruits at 80% Acid Binding – Eat And Drink These Fruits Apricots, avocados, bananas, fresh dates, fresh figs, currants, gooseberries grapes, grapefruits guavas, kumquats, nectarines, pears, persimmons, quince

5. Fruits at 73% Acid Binding – Still Fruits To Eat And Drink Apples, organs, peaches, pomegranate, raspberries, sour grapes, strawberries

6. Fruits at 67% Acid Binding – Still Neutralizes Acids, Eat And Drink This fruit Cherries

Fruits To Concentrate On

These are the fruits you should concentrate on eating. Also, eat them every day, if possible, fresh lemon juice in the morning, watermelon during the day.

You can see which fruits give you the best acid binding effects and eating and drinking them 80% of your overall food intake will convert your body over to an Alkaline body.

Here is another rule. If you eat an acid food like meat, which is a 13% and an alkaline binding food that is 80 - 100%, you can offset the meat's acids. Don't eat fruit at the same time you your meals. They use different enzymes in your stomach for digestion.

Drinking fruit juices help to bring vitamins and minerals quickly into your blood. Minerals are the key to keeping your body alkaline. Keeping an alkaline body, helps you keep away disease and will strengthen your cardiovascular system.

Juices have antibacterial action and contain digestive enzymes that help you to digest protein and fat. Because of the vitamins, minerals, digestive enzymes, pure water, and nutrients that fresh juices have, they have the power to cleanse your body of toxic wastes, lower your blood pressure, and make your heart stronger.

Try to use organic fruit when making your juice. It is better to make your own juices, since most bottled juice contains no life force or natural live enzymes. Drink the juices soon after you juice them. If you want, put them in a thermos for later in the day. If you have no choice but to use store juices, get them in bottles instead of plastic. Plastic bottles leach out toxic chemicals that are used in their production.

Here Are Some Juices to Drink.

Apple juice

Drink at least two glasses of this juice every day. Apple juice has a high level of minerals and vitamins, which make it ideal for making your body alkaline.

Apricot – berry juice

Mix equal parts of apricot and berry juice and add a little honey to taste. Drink one cup in the morning. Place the other two glasses into a thermos and drink one more glass at noon and one at dinner.

Berries

Blackberries – help cleanse the blood and are good for constipation. They help a weak kidney and are filled with antioxidants, which fight plaque buildup in your arteries.

Cherry juice

Cherry juice is a powerful drink. Because it has so many minerals, it will make your body more alkaline by neutralize acid waste in the blood, in the lymph liquid and wherever it goes. It will also help in keeping you regular. Cherries are good blood cleansers and help the liver and kidney.

Grape Juice

Add grape juice to other juices like apple to give it a different flavor. When juicing apples, you can add a few handfuls of grapes to create a new mixture. Grapes have a high content of natural sugar and can give you a quick energy lift. They contain a high level of minerals and have B vitamins.

You can use bottled juices, since some fruits have a short season and in a bottle, you can drink it any time. Use the darker grape drinks, because of their high anti-oxidant nutrients

Grapes help to regulate and increase your metabolism. A low metabolism will cause you to gain weight, and a high metabolism will help you burn food quicker and get you tired sooner.

Because of its mineral content, it helps to build your blood and to stimulate your liver to increase its cleansing abilities. The color of fruit juices often tells you what part of the body it is good for. Red grape juice helps build your blood.

Lemon Juice

Lemon juice is one of the best juices you can drink to help detoxify your liver. It contains many minerals, which will eliminate acid waste. Lemon juice will help constipation, liver disorders, reduce mucus accumulation, improve digestion, reduce infections, and help to clear skin disorders.

One way to use lemon juice is to squeeze the juice of one lemon into 8 oz. of water and drink it first thing in the morning. You can also carry unsweetened lemon water in a thermos and drink it during the day.

Melons

Melon juice is almost the perfect food in that it has many vitamins and minerals. It is most helpful with constipation and kidney and skin disorders. Melons and Cantaloupes are high in vitamin A, C and have many other minerals. Do not eat them with other fruits or juices. But, you can eat them with watermelon or other types of melons.

Orange and grapefruit

Prepare half and half of orange and grapefruit juice, using a hand juicer. The flavor is extremely tasty. The combination of these two fresh fruits will give you a powerful start in the morning. They will give you a vitamin C boost with plenty of flavonoids and minerals.

These combined fruits will cleanse your intestinal tract, help in blood disorders, liver disorders, and lung disorders.

Orange and lemon juice

Mix 3 parts of orange juice with one part lemon juice. Add a little water and honey and put into a thermos. Drink the juice all day long.

Pineapples

Pineapple juice increases male potency, reduces menstrual cycle issues, and strengthens muscles and tissues. It reduces body acidity and excess bile and strengthens the heart.

Pineapple juice is another excellent juice to use frequently. Its high potassium helps to keep your brain nerve transmission active. Its health value comes from the enzyme bromelain that it contains. Bromelain helps keep body fluid balance and neutral; it moves an acid body to neutral and an alkaline one to neutral. It stimulates the pancreas to release its hormones.

And, it has been found useful for coughs and sore throats. For some people, pineapple juice affects the throat making it feel scratchy.

Pineapples contain many vitamins and minerals. They contain Papain, which helps to digest protein. Pineapples are useful when you have excess mucus, digestive problems, intestinal worms, and constipation.

Pomegranate

Pomegranate juice is one of the best juices to get yourself back to health and for helping you regain your manhood. Pomegranate juice controls bile and phlegm, increases hemoglobin and purifies blood, and improves appetite, and settles upset stomachs.

It restores and sharpens memory, and is effective in urinary issues. It is helpful in many diseases, since it neutralizes body acids. It will cure nose bleed by placing a couple drops in each nose. It is excellent for reducing fever. Drinking half a glass or more twice a day will help you reduce high blood pressure.

Watermelon

Here is another excellent fruit to eat. Watermelon juice can be obtained by simply eating raw watermelon, since it is 98%

distilled water. Its use helps cleanse the kidney and bladder, since it is a diuretic – removes excess fluids from the body. You can chew on the seeds as you eat watermelon to get extra zinc and vitamin E.

Watermelon juice tones your body, prevents heat stroke, normalizes high blood pressure, and strengthens your heart and brain. It helps to cure jaundice and spleen enlargement. It improves digestion, cures chronic headaches, controls nausea and vomiting, calms the nerves, and is a mild laxative.

Eating watermelon in the morning to get its juice will help you remove nightly accumulated toxins through your urine. This will you restore kidney function.

10: The Best Whole Fruits That Make You Alkaline

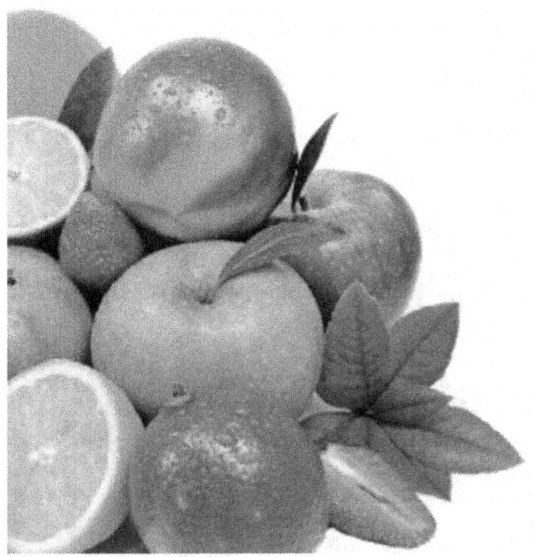

Fruits

Because fruits are naturally grown from the soil, they pull minerals from the ground, and they are a great source of nutrients for you, if the soil is heavy with minerals. Because of these minerals and other nutrients, fruits have amazing curative effects, when they are eaten raw. In some cases, it is better to cook them for their healing effects.

Fruits contain a variety of nutrients that are necessary for maintaining life. Each nutrient has its function in your body. Many of these functions are known, and many are not. Here is a list of some of the main known nutrients.

- Minerals

- Antioxidants
- Vitamins
- Fiber
- Natural water
- Enzymes
- Phytonutrients
- Unknown chemicals

Minerals

There are many minerals and vitamins that are classified as antioxidants. These are vitamins A, C, E, and selenium. Other antioxidants are bioflavonoids, carotenoids, and isoflavones. Vegetables have antioxidants, minerals and nutrients that cure disease. Your body uses these antioxidants to stop the formation of deadly diseases in your body.

Eat fruits between meals and alternate between drinking them as juice and eating them whole.

Bananas

Eat only one to two banana a day. Bananas have the phytochemicals fructoOligosaccharides, which feeds the good bacterial in your colon. By feeding the good bacteria, you prevent the bad bacteria from overtaking the colon and producing toxic acids.

Bananas are high in potassium and fiber. They are a good source of Folate, vitamin C, and B-6. Bananas contain practically no sodium. However, sodium is one of the top nutrients to consume. But, only the sodium in fruits and vegetables is what your body needs.

Apples

Apples are high in soluble fiber, with the skin containing small amounts of beta carotene. They contain vitamin C, potassium and some iron. Apples in the morning provide fiber and pectin, which helps to clean out your colon.

You can also eat dried apples, but most nutrients are lost in the drying process except iron and fiber.

Apricots

Apricots have a short season, and that is why you see a lot of dried apricots for sale. Eat apricots in season. They are high in beta carotene, iron, potassium, and vitamin C. They also are high in fiber.

Dried apricots are more nutritious than fresh, since the nutrients are more concentrated. The major problem with dried apricots is that they are dried with sulfur dioxide and this creates more acid and health issues in your stomach.

There are some dried apricots that use low sulfur dioxide and some that use no sulfur dioxide.

Avocados

Avocado is a fruit. It is one of the fruits that is highest in mono-unsaturated fatty acid, omega-9, which is a good fat. Most avocado fat consists of 60 - 75% omega-9. It also contains vitamin E, folic acid, fiber and many other nutrients. Omega-9 is an important omega to consume, and few foods contain this nutrient in this high concentration.

Berries

Berries, blackberries, raspberries, strawberries are high in fiber and antioxidants. The deeper that colors – red, blue, and black - the more antioxidants they have. Antioxidants combine with free radicals in your body to deactivate them.

Free radicals are now considered the molecular ions that cause the most damage in your body. Neutralizing them is one of your first priorities.

Cantaloupes

Cantaloupe is one of the best fruits to eat. It has a high source of antioxidants, vitamin C, and beta carotene. It is also high in fiber. Eat cantaloupes only with other melons and do not eat it with other fruits. The stomach enzymes necessary to digest cantaloupes are different from other fruits and the stomach concentrates on digesting similar types of fruit at a time.

Cherries

Cherries are high in vitamin C, pectin, potassium and soluble fiber. Eating cherries and their juices will help you maintain regular bowel movement, when consumed between meals.

Figs

Figs are high in fiber and can be eaten fresh or dried. They are a good source of magnesium, potassium, calcium, iron, Vitamin B6 and Folate. Because they are high in sugar, their stickiness can contribute to tooth decay. So when you eat fresh figs, rinse your mouth out with water afterwards.

Eating figs with other fruits high in Vitamin C will increase the absorption of iron. Figs are highly recommended for people who have issues with constipation.

Grapefruits

Grapefruit has a unique type of soluble fiber call galacturonic acid. They are high in vitamin C and potassium. They are a good source of Folate, iron, calcium, beta carotene, and minerals.

They should not be eaten, if you are on blood-thinning drugs. When taken with drugs they tend to enhance the effect of the drug or other vitamins taken. Some people are allergic to grapefruit.

Grapes

Grapes are high in pectin and bioflavonoids. They are a good source of iron, potassium and vitamin C. They provide for an excellent snack between meals. One problem with them is they are highly treated with pesticides.

Guavas

Guavas are high in lycopene due its red flesh. It is an excellent source vitamin C and other nutrients. It is a good source of pectin and other soluble fiber. It contains a good amount of iron and potassium. The outer skin is edible. It can be mixed with other fruits, but eating it alone is better, since it will digest faster and provide you with its nutrients quickly.

Lemons

Lemons are a great source of vitamin C and provide plenty of bioflavonoids and antioxidants. Using the juice of one lemon in the morning with 6+ oz. of water is a great way to help cleanse the liver and the kidney.

Limes like lemons are great source of vitamin C, bioflavonoids and antioxidants. It also can be used as lime juice in the morning to help the detox process take place in the morning.

Mangos

Mangos are an excellent source of beta carotene, vitamin C

and fiber. It contains vitamin E, niacin, potassium and iron. Mangos have been associated with a decrease in breast cancer when eaten regularly. Use it to make morning smoothies.

Nectarines

Nectarines contain plenty of beta carotene, potassium, vitamin C vitamin A. It's a great source of soluble fiber.

Oranges

Oranges are excellent for vitamin C, beta carotene, Folate, thiamin and potassium. Combine the juice of one or two oranges with one lemon in 8 oz. of water to get your morning going.

Peaches

Peaches are a good source of vitamin A and pectin fiber. It has useful amount of vitamin C, potassium, antioxidants.

Pears

Pears are a good source of vitamin C, Folate, and fiber. Pears when in season provide for an excellent snack. They tend to ripen fast, so they need to be eaten as they turn yellow. Canned pears lose most of their vitamin C value, as do all other fruit that are canned.

Papayas

Papayas contain the protein digestive enzyme papain. Papain is similar to pepsin, which is the digestive enzyme found in our stomach. They also contain a good amount of vitamin A, beta-carotene, potassium, and vitamin C.

As you can see many of the fruits contain a lot of vitamin C, potassium, beta carotene, antioxidants, bioflavonoids, and fiber. So these are important nutrients, which your body uses during the detoxification process and body building.

Your body also uses these nutrients to neutralize acids in your cells so that they can continue to function properly and stop the formation of disease.

11: The Best Vegetables That Make You Alkaline

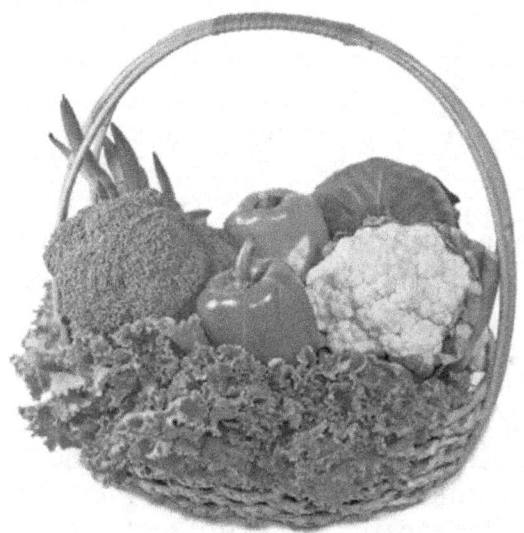

Did you know that there are certain vegetables you should be eating to make your body more alkaline? These vegetables have the chemicals and elements that transform tissues, cells, and organs into an alkaline condition. This is one of their basic functions.

Vegetables and their juices also have curative powers for preventing and eliminating illness and disease.

Vegetables

Phytochemicals are all the chemicals that exist in vegetables and fruits. There are so many phytochemicals that scientists have yet to investigate and learn about all of them.

You should be eating vegetables of all colors. Use them mostly in raw form to get the benefits of the fiber they have, which will help keep your colon clean. In the raw form, they contain natural enzymes that help you to digest them. And, in raw form they contain the most vitamins and minerals.

If you cook them in a little water and cook them only for up to 4 minutes or so to keep them firm. Cooking them too long causes them to lose nutrients that you need for your general health.

Always eat vegetables with your main protein or carbohydrate.

This provides the fiber needed to digest and move this protein or carbohydrate through your body and especially through your colon.

Cooking Vegetables

Vegetables can be stir-fried, steamed, sautéed, or grilled. It is good to eat vegetables in a variety of ways, since different nutrients are available based on how they are cooked. By eating vegetable prepared in a different way in a meal, you stand to get the best possible variety of nutrients into your body. When stir-frying them, use coconut oil since this oil can take a higher heat before it starts to produce free radicals.

Here are some of the best vegetables to eat raw. There are only a few vegetables that you should not eat raw.

- Bamboo shoots
- Green beans
- Cauliflower
- Collards, Mustard greens
- Chervil
- Chicory
- Corn
- Watercress
- Daikon radish
- Eggplant

- Escarole
- Fennel
- Leek, Shallot
- Lettuce- romaine, butter, red curly
- Mushrooms
- Okra
- Peas
- Bell peppers
- Potato
- Rhubarb
- Rutabaga
- String beans
- Squash, summer, winter, zucchini
- Sweet potato
- Yam

12: Final Thoughts

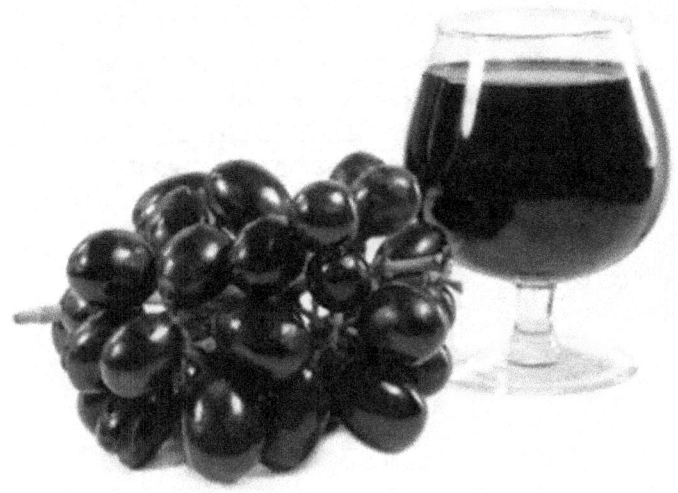

Cleansing the colon and the blood is the first thing you should do when you are moving in a new health direction. And, if your health is not so good, then it is necessary for you to this type of cleanse.

Because the colon is central to your body's health, any improvement you make in its function multiplies throughout your body. After you do a colon cleanse, then you can think about doing a kidney cleanse and after that a liver cleanse.

The very center of your overall health and the health your will have later in life is determined by the food you eat now. Because the food industry is not geared to providing you with the type of nutrition, your body really needs, you have to take charge of what foods you will prepare and eat.

The food industry is based on profit, quick food, packaged food, and preserving food. All of these processes require the use of chemical additives that shorten your life by creating disease. Your life will further be shortening, if you start using drugs for these diseases.

Increasing the use of fruits and vegetables is the direction of health. Eating refined foods is the direction of sickness. It is the toxins and the lack of fiber in processed foods that make you sick. It is the alteration of food that your body has a problem with. In many cases, your body can't recognize the changes in these foods, so it treats them as toxins and stores them throughout your body as fat or toxic waste.

These toxins affect your DNA and provide new information to your genes on how to make up your body, when they create replacement cells.

13: About The Author And Other Resources

Get one of my best kindle books *free* below:

http://www.natural-remedies-thatwork.com

Rudy Silva is a natural nutritional consultant educated in the United States in Nutrition and Physics. He is a graduate from San Jose State University in California. He is author of 45 other books on natural remedies. He has authored a newsletter in natural remedies for over 10 years.

Resource page

Here are some of the other kindle e-books about natural remedies that have been written by this author. You can see the entire list at:

http://tinyurl.com/b2f7wd3

Acne Remedies

- Best natural acne treatments: Acne facial
- Effective Acne Treatments That Work

Constipation Remedies
- The Best Constipation Remedies
- Best Constipated Women Natural Cures
- How To Relieve Constipation With Fruits

Essential Fatty Acids

- Taking The Mystery Out Of Essential Fatty acids

- Amazing Fish Oil Benefits Revealed
- Omega 3 and 6 Mystery Exposed

Nutrition Remedies

- Updated Version - Secret Diet And Nutrition
- Secret Healthy Fruit Practices Revealed
- Fast Healing Juice Nutrition Therapy: Nutrition Tips 3
- Fantastic Alkaline Fruit Benefits Revealed
- Calcium (Discover How To Use Calcium To Avoid Devastating Diseases)
- Magnesium Nutrition Revealed
- Best Nutrition Health Practices
- Potassium Health Secrets Revealed
- Phosphorus, The Best Brain Food
- A Sodium Diet (What You Must Know About Sodium)
- Vegetables and Vegetable Juice Cures
- Alkaline Body: How to Change an Acid Body into an Alkaline body

Stomach Remedies
- Acid Reflux: Fast and Easy Cures For Acid Reflux
- Asthma Treatment Cures With Remedies
- How To Do Natural Colon Cleansing
- Gastrointestinal Digestion Secrets Revealed

Misc Remedies

- Natural Hair Loss Treatment: Women And Men
- Effective Natural Hemorrhoids Treatment
- Iron Deficiency Anemia
- Secrets To Understanding Behavior
- Fast Acting Ear Infection Remedies
- Best Behavior Secrets Revealed That Can Change Your Personality
- What Is A Hiatus Hernia

- Best Varicose Vein Treatments?
- Make Shampoos At Home Using Natural Ingredients:Discover recipes for quality natural hair shampoos
- How To Fix Your Thyroid Problems: Discover Hidden Ideas That Fix Your Thyroid

Minerals

- Calcium and Magnesium Magic Body Benefits Revealed
- The Magic of Sodium, Calcium and Magnesium
- Create an Alkaline Body with Potassium and Sodium: Eliminate a Potassium Deficiency
- Calcium and Phosphorus Foods: Deficiency or Excesses in These Minerals Cause Bone and Brain Power Loss
- Chlorine The Body Detoxifier (With water, chlorine will clean your body of toxins and pathogens)

Men's Health

- Best Impotence Health Diet

Weight loss

- Ten (10) Day Quick Success Weight Loss Program: A new approach to losing weight by changing your eating habits for life
- Discover Secret Anti-Aging Juice & Tonic Recipes: Unique Juices And Tonics That Create Beauty And Youth

To see all the kindle books written by this author, go to this the Authors Profile Page or this URL: http://tinyurl.com/b2f7wd3

If you need support or want to promote any of his e-books, please contact him at rss41@yahoo.com and expect a reply within 24 hours. He looks forward to hearing from you and is happy to help you understand his material on natural and nutritional health.

Give a Review

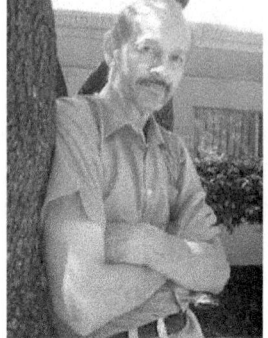

And, don't for get to give a review for this e-book at Amazon so that others can gain the benefits of what is in this e-book. To you, for losing weight, creating better health and more happiness in your life,

Rudy S Silva

www.ingramcontent.com/pod-product-compliance
Lightning Source LLC
Chambersburg PA
CBHW070608290526
45790CB00002B/834